# ALZHEIMER'S DISEASE DIET COOKBOOK

Nutrient-Rich Recipes For Brain Health, Memory Support, And Cognitive Function Enhancement

## DR ELIAN GRIFFIN

Copyright © [Dr. Elian Griffin] [2024]. All rights reserved.

Without the publisher's prior written consent, no portion of this publication may be copied, distributed, or transmitted in any way, including by photocopying, recording, or other mechanical or electronic means, with the exception of brief quotations used in all critical reviews.

# DISCLAIMER

The nutritional recommendations and recipes in this book are meant solely for informative reasons. They are not meant to replace the counsel, diagnosis, or care of a qualified medical expert. If you have any doubts about a medical condition or dietary requirements, you should always see your physician or another trained healthcare expert.

All reasonable efforts have been taken by the author and publisher to ensure that the information contained in this book is correct as of the date of publication. Recommendations may alter, though, as medical knowledge is always changing. When using any of the recipes or instructions found here, the user assumes all liability and assumes no risk, whether personal or otherwise. People who have certain dietary requirements or medical issues should speak with a healthcare provider for personalized guidance. The given recipes are only ideas; you may need to adjust them to suit your own nutritional needs, tastes, and tolerances.

When you use this book, you agree to release the publisher, the author, and their representatives from any liability for any claims, damages, liabilities, costs, or expenditures resulting from your use of the book.

# TABLE OF CONTENTS

## CHAPTER ONE .................................................................................. 13
### ALZHEIMER'S DISEASE DIET INTRODUCTION ............................................ 13
- WHAT IS ALZHEIMER'S AND HOW DOES DIET AFFECT IT? ................. 13
- THE ROLE OF DIET IN TREATING ALZHEIMER'S SYMPTOMS............... 14
- HOW USING THIS COOKBOOK CAN HELP YOU L VE A BETTER .......... 15
- SUMMARY OF TYPICAL NUTRITIONAL ISSUES ALZHEIMER'S ............. 16
- A REMARK ON THE SIGNIFICANCE OF SEEKING ADVICE FROM.......... 17

## CHAPTER TWO .................................................................................. 19
### FUNDAMENTALS OF ALZHEIMER'S DISEASE DIET . ................................... 19
- RECOGNIZING THE NUTRITIONAL REQUIREMENTS FOR BRAIN HEALTH................................................................................. 19
- ITEMS TO ADD AND SUBTRACT FROM YOUR ALZHEIMER'S DIET ...... 20
- HYDRATION'S SIGNIFICANCE AND EFFECT ON COGNITIVE ............... 21
- HOW NUTRITION CAN HELP PROMOTE GENERAL HEALTH............... 23
- ADVICE ON HOW TO MODIFY RECIPES FOR DIETARY ....................... 24

## CHAPTER THREE ............................................................................... 27
### CRUCIAL ELEMENTS FOR MENTAL WELL-BEING ..................................... 27
- ANTIOXIDANTS' FUNCTION IN BRAIN PROTECTION.......................... 27
- THE VALUE AND SOURCES OF OMEGA-3 FATTY ACIDS ..................... 28
- VITAMIN AND MINERAL NEEDS FOR INDIVIDUALS WITH .................. 29
- THE IMPACT OF PROTEIN CONSUMPTION ON BRAIN ACTIVITY ........ 30
- FIBER INCLUSION FOR IMPROVED DIGESTIVE HEALTH AND ............. 31

## CHAPTER FOUR ................................................................................. 33
### STRATEGIES FOR MEAL PLANNING ....................................................... 33
- EASY WAYS TO PLAN MEALS FOR CAREGIVERS................................. 33

- PREPARING EASY-TO-PREPARE, BALANCED MEALS ............................ 34
- CHANGING PORTION SIZES TO SUIT DIFFERENT APPETITES ............... 36
- SOME ADVICE FOR KEEPING MEAL SCHEDULES CONSISTENT ........... 37
- INCLUDING VARIATION TO BOOST NUTRITIOUS CONSUMPTION ....... 38

SIMPLE AND FAST BREAKFAST RECIPES ................................................. 40
- HEALTHY SMOOTHIE RECIPES TO GET YOU STARTED FAST ............... 40
- EASY VARIATIONS FOR OATMEAL AND PORRIDGE ............................ 41
- EGG-BASED RECIPES PACKED WITH VITAL NUTRIENTS ...................... 42
- BREAKFAST IDEAS THAT CAN BE APPLIED TO VARIOUS DIETS ........... 43
- SOME ADVICE FOR PROMOTING BREAKFAST CONSUMPTION .......... 44

HEALTHY LUNCH AND DINNER SUGGESTIONS ..................................... 45
- EASY-TO-DIGEST ONE-POT DINNERS .................................................. 45
- RICH IN NUTRIENT SOUPS AND STEWS .............................................. 46
- VEGETABLE-HEAVY SALADS WITH COMPONENTS THAT .................... 47
- DINNERTIME MAIN DISHES PACKED WITH PROTEIN ......................... 48
- HOW TO ADJUST TEXTURES TO MAKE THEM EASIER TO ................... 49

SNACKS AND DRINKS TO REFUEL AND STAY HYDRATED ....................... 51
- OPTIONS FOR HEALTHFUL SNACKS TO KEEP YOUR ENERGY LEVELS UP ............................................................................................................. 51
- DRINKS THAT REHYDRATE AND PROMOTE COGNITIVE ..................... 52
- HOW TO MAKE HEALTHY SNACKS AT HOME ..................................... 53
- SNACK IDEAS TO CONTROL YOUR APPETITE IN BETWEEN ................ 55
- REASONS WHY MINDFUL EATING IS IMPORTANT FOR ...................... 56

CHAPTER FIVE ........................................................................................ 59

RECIPES FOR SPECIAL OCCASIONS AND HOLIDAYS ............................... 59

FESTIVE RECIPES ........................................................................ 59
HOW TO MODIFY TRADITIONAL DISHES FOR DIETARY NEEDS .......... 60
DESSERTS WITH BRAIN-BOOSTING INGREDIENTS .............................. 61
CREATING A COMFORTING MEAL ENVIRONMENT FOR HOLIDAYS .... 62
TIPS FOR INCLUDING ALZHEIMER'S PATIENTS IN MEAL PREPARATION ................................................................................................................ 64

# CHAPTER SIX ............................................................................................. 67
## COOKING TRICKS AND STRATEGIES FOR SENIORS ................................ 67
SETTING UP THE KITCHEN TO MAKE MEAL PREPARATION EASIER .... 67
FLEXIBLE KITCHEN UTENSILS AND APPLIANCES ................................ 68
HOW TO BE PATIENT WHEN FACING COOKING DIFFICULTIES ........... 69
ADVICE FOR PROMOTING SELF-SUFFICIENCY IN MEAL ...................... 70
SAFETY STEPS TO AVOID MISHAPS IN THE KITCHEN ......................... 71

# CHAPTER SEVEN ...................................................................................... 73
## TAKING CARE OF EATING CHALLENGES AND DIETARY ADJUSTMENTS .. 73
RECOGNIZING TYPICAL EATING CHALLENGES IN ALZHEIMER'S PATIENTS ................................................................................................ 73
HOW TO HANDLE TASTE AND APPETITE SHIFTS ............................... 74
ADVICE FOR ENCOURAGING SATISFYING MEAL EXPERIENCES .......... 76
MODIFYING RECIPES TO ADDRESS CHEWING AND ........................... 77
COLLABORATING WITH MEDICAL EXPERTS TO PROVIDE ................... 78

# CHAPTER EIGHT ....................................................................................... 80
## COMMON QUESTIONS AND EXTENSIVE ANSWERS ............................. 80
TAKING CARE OF NUTRITIONAL ISSUES PARTICULAR TO ALZHEIMER'S PATIENTS ................................................................................................ 80
HOW TO MANAGE NUTRITIONAL ADJUSTMENTS AS ......................... 81

STRATEGIES FOR HANDLING WEIGHT GAIN OR LOSS ........................ 82

RECOGNIZING SUPPLEMENTS' SIGNIFICANCE IN ALZHEIMER'S ......... 84

RESPONSES TO COMMON QUESTIONS CONCERNING THE ................ 85

## ABOUT THE BOOK

Understanding the impact of nutrition on cognitive function is crucial, as diet plays a pivotal role in managing symptoms and improving overall quality of life. The Alzheimer's Disease Diet Cookbook is an indispensable resource for caregivers and individuals navigating the complexities of managing Alzheimer's disease through nutrition. Alzheimer's disease is a progressive neurodegenerative condition that presents unique challenges that can be influenced by dietary choices.

This cookbook begins by explaining the basic principles of Alzheimer's disease and the significant impact that diet can have on its course. It highlights the significance of customized nutrition plans in reducing symptoms like memory loss and cognitive decline. It also walks caregivers and patients through the complexities of meal planning, making sure that dietary requirements are satisfied while taking individual preferences and limitations into account.

The scientific basis of the cookbook is reinforced by an extensive examination of the critical nutrients for cognitive health. Each nutrient's role in brain function is explained in detail, ranging from antioxidants' protective effects on brain cells to the importance of omega-3 fatty acids and essential vitamins. Caregivers can also benefit from practical advice on how to incorporate these nutrients into regular meals.

Along with providing practical solutions for caregivers, the cookbook promotes balanced, simple-to-prepare meals that are tailored to varying appetites and dietary needs, guaranteeing consistency in nutritional support. Recipes are not only meant to nourish but also to stimulate appetite and encourage regular eating habits, which are critical for maintaining overall health.

The importance of maintaining a sufficient fluid intake through homemade snacks and hydrating beverages is emphasized; along with the role that hydration plays in cognitive function. Practical solutions and empathetic discussion of strategies for managing eating difficulties, such as taste changes or swallowing difficulties enable caregivers to serve meals that are enjoyable and nourishing.

The cookbook is a valuable resource for navigating the nutritional complexities associated with Alzheimer's disease because it addresses common concerns and provides detailed FAQs. It also emphasizes the importance of collaborating with healthcare professionals and emphasizes the need for individualized dietary guidance tailored to the specific needs and progression of Alzheimer's disease.

# CHAPTER ONE

## ALZHEIMER'S DISEASE DIET INTRODUCTION

## WHAT IS ALZHEIMER'S AND HOW DOES DIET AFFECT IT?

Alzheimer's disease is a neurological condition that worsens over time and impairs thinking, memory, and behavior. It is caused by plaques and tangles building up in the brain, which interfere with neuronal communication and cause cognitive decline. Although there is no known cure for Alzheimer's disease, research indicates that diet may be very important in controlling the disease's course and symptoms.

On the other hand, diets high in saturated fats and processed foods have been linked to an increased risk of cognitive decline.

Certain nutrients, such as antioxidants found in fruits and vegetables, omega-3 fatty acids from fish, and vitamin E from nuts and seeds, have been linked to brain health and may help reduce inflammation and oxidative stress in the brain.

This cookbook aims to provide recipes that are rich in nutrients that are beneficial to the brain and that are both enjoyable and accessible for patients and caregivers. A balanced diet that includes a variety of nutrient-dense foods can support overall health and may help delay the onset or progression of Alzheimer's disease.

## THE ROLE OF DIET IN TREATING ALZHEIMER'S SYMPTOMS

Because it can impact mood, behavior, and cognitive function, nutrition is an important part of managing Alzheimer's symptoms. People with Alzheimer's disease frequently have changes in appetite, taste perception, and meal preparation skills, which can result in malnutrition and further deterioration in health.

Healthy weight management, provision of vital nutrients for brain function, and support for general well-being can all be achieved with a well-planned diet. Antioxidant-rich foods (berries, leafy greens, etc.) can help shield brain cells from damage, and omega-3 fatty acids (found in fish, such as salmon and flaxseeds) are important for brain health and may enhance memory and cognitive function.

Caregivers can make sure their loved ones receive enough nutrition to support their physical and cognitive health by focusing on nutrient-dense ingredients and simple cooking techniques.

This cookbook is intended to provide wholesome and delicious recipes that are simple to prepare and appealing to individuals with Alzheimer's disease.

## HOW USING THIS COOKBOOK CAN HELP YOU LIVE A BETTER LIFE

Meal preparation can be difficult for caregivers, especially when dealing with dietary limitations and changing tastes. This cookbook for those on an Alzheimer's disease diet strives to improve the quality of life for patients and caregivers by offering a variety of wholesome and practical meal options.

This cookbook makes meal preparation easier for Alzheimer's patients by providing a range of simple-to-follow recipes that are adapted to meet their specific nutritional needs. All of the recipes are made to be tasty, easy to chew and swallow, and full of vital nutrients that support overall well-being and brain health.

Sharing meals with family and friends can create a sense of routine and familiarity, which is comforting for people with Alzheimer's disease, this cookbook not only provides nourishing meals but also promotes social interaction and engagement during mealtime, which can help reduce feelings of isolation and improve mood.

## SUMMARY OF TYPICAL NUTRITIONAL ISSUES ALZHEIMER'S PATIENTS FACE

Alzheimer's patients frequently experience several dietary difficulties that can affect their nutritional intake and general health. These difficulties can include altered appetites and taste preferences, trouble chewing and swallowing, and difficulties organizing and preparing meals.

As the disease worsens, people may also have memory and cognitive problems that make it difficult for them to identify hunger and thirst signals or to remember to eat regularly. To make sure that their loved ones are getting enough nutrition, caregivers may need to keep a close eye on their food intake.

Caretakers can support brain health and overall well-being by focusing on foods that are rich in antioxidants, vitamins, and minerals.

This cookbook addresses these common dietary challenges and offers recipes that are simple to prepare, nutrient-dense, and appealing to individuals with Alzheimer's disease.

## A REMARK ON THE SIGNIFICANCE OF SEEKING ADVICE FROM MEDICAL EXPERTS

Although the Alzheimer's disease diet cookbook offers helpful dietary advice and recipes, patients, and caregivers must speak with medical professionals before making any big dietary adjustments.

A person's medical history, present state of health, and dietary preferences can all be taken into account when making personalized recommendations from healthcare professionals like doctors, dietitians, and nutritionists. They can also help with specific nutritional needs and concerns like managing medications that may interact with certain foods or supplements.

In close collaboration with medical professionals, caregivers can help optimize health outcomes and improve the quality of life for patients and caregivers alike by making sure their loved ones receive the best care and support for managing Alzheimer's disease through nutrition.

# CHAPTER TWO

## FUNDAMENTALS OF ALZHEIMER'S DISEASE DIET

### RECOGNIZING THE NUTRITIONAL REQUIREMENTS FOR BRAIN HEALTH

A balanced diet rich in essential nutrients is necessary for the brain to function at its best. Antioxidants such as vitamins C and E help shield brain cells from damage caused by free radicals; omega-3 fatty acids, found in walnuts and salmon, are important for cognitive function and can help reduce inflammation in the brain; and B vitamins, especially folate and B12, support nerve function and help prevent cognitive decline. Keeping the brain healthy is crucial, especially for those who have Alzheimer's disease.

Dark leafy greens like spinach and kale are rich in antioxidants and vitamin K, which support brain health by aiding in blood clotting and cognitive function. Whole grains like oatmeal and brown rice provide a steady supply of energy to the brain, helping to maintain focus and mental clarity throughout the day. A diet focused on brain health should also include plenty of fruits and vegetables, as they provide vitamins, minerals, and fiber essential for overall well-being.

Choosing natural, whole foods that nourish the brain and support cognitive function over time is the key to improving brain health through nutrition. Processed foods high in sugars and unhealthy fats can exacerbate symptoms of Alzheimer's disease by causing inflammation and oxidative stress in the brain.

## ITEMS TO ADD AND SUBTRACT FROM YOUR ALZHEIMER'S DIET

Including a wide range of vibrant fruits and vegetables, which offer antioxidants that help shield brain cells from damage, is an important part of an Alzheimer's diet. Berries, like strawberries and blueberries, are especially helpful because of their high levels of antioxidants called flavonoids, which have been linked to enhanced cognitive function.

Moderate consumption of healthy fats, such as those found in avocados, nuts, and olive oil, is important for brain health because they support communication between brain cells and preserve the integrity of brain cell membranes. Fatty fish, like salmon, trout, and sardines, are rich in omega-3 fatty acids, which are important for maintaining cognitive function and have anti-inflammatory properties.

On the other hand, foods high in trans and saturated fats, like processed snacks, fried foods, and fatty meat cuts, should be limited because they raise cholesterol and can lead to cognitive decline. You should also cut back on refined sugars and carbohydrates because they can cause blood sugar spikes and crashes, which can have a long-term negative effect on brain health.

## HYDRATION'S SIGNIFICANCE AND EFFECT ON COGNITIVE PROCESS

Proper hydration helps ensure that the brain receives enough oxygen and nutrients through the bloodstream, supporting overall brain health.

Dehydration can lead to confusion, dizziness, and fatigue, which can exacerbate symptoms of cognitive decline. This is especially important for people with Alzheimer's disease.

Aim for at least eight glasses of water per day, or more if you live in a hot climate or participate in physical activity that increases sweating. Urine color can be a helpful indicator of hydration status; pale yellow or clear urine usually indicates adequate hydration. Water is the best choice for staying hydrated, but other fluids like herbal teas and broths can also contribute to daily fluid intake.

Establishing routine and providing fluids throughout the day can be beneficial for Alzheimer's patients who may forget to drink water regularly. Caregivers should keep an eye on the patient's hydration levels and be alert to any symptoms of dehydration, such as dark urine or dry mouth, to ensure the patient's best possible cognitive function and general well-being.

## HOW NUTRITION CAN HELP PROMOTE GENERAL HEALTH

Eating a variety of nutrient-dense foods helps maintain a healthy weight, which is important for managing chronic conditions like diabetes and heart disease that can coexist with Alzheimer's. A healthy weight also supports mobility and reduces the risk of falls, which can be particularly important for older adults. A well-balanced diet not only supports brain health but also contributes to overall well-being for individuals with Alzheimer's disease.

In addition to providing the energy required for everyday tasks, a healthy diet can stabilize blood sugar levels, prevent irritability or confusion caused by hunger or low energy, improve mood, and reduce behavioral symptoms associated with Alzheimer's disease, such as aggression and agitation.

A pleasant and relaxed atmosphere with few distractions and enough time for eating can also support digestion and nutrient absorption. Social aspects of mealtime, such as dining with family or friends, can improve the overall dining experience and foster feelings of connection and well-being. Caregivers are essential in ensuring that people with Alzheimer's disease receive enough nutrition and have a positive dining experience that supports their overall well-being.

## ADVICE ON HOW TO MODIFY RECIPES FOR DIETARY RESTRICTIONS

Incorporating a range of herbs and spices to enhance flavor without relying on salt, which may need to be restricted for individuals with heart disease or hypertension, can be difficult, but it's crucial for those with Alzheimer's disease who may have particular nutritional needs or food sensitivities. Begin by concentrating on whole, unprocessed foods that are naturally gluten-free or low in sodium and sugars.

When adjusting recipes, think about substituting ingredients that satisfy dietary requirements without sacrificing flavor or texture. For instance, instead of using wheat flour for gluten-free baking, try using almond or coconut flour, or replace sugar in desserts with unsweetened applesauce or mashed bananas. Try different cooking techniques, like grilling, steaming, or baking, to cut down on the amount of fat and oil needed while maintaining flavor and nutrients.

Be proactive and creative in the kitchen to ensure that people with Alzheimer's disease enjoy tasty and nutritious meals that support their overall health and well-being. Speak with a registered dietitian or nutritionist for personalized guidance on modifying recipes to meet specific dietary needs or preferences. They can offer expert advice on ingredient substitutions, portion sizes, and meal planning strategies that optimize nutrition while accommodating individual tastes and dietary restrictions.

# CHAPTER THREE

## CRUCIAL ELEMENTS FOR MENTAL WELL-BEING

## ANTIOXIDANTS' FUNCTION IN BRAIN PROTECTION

Strong antioxidants, such as vitamin C, vitamin E, and flavonoids found in fruits and vegetables like spinach and kale, neutralize free radicals, and unstable molecules that can damage cells and contribute to cognitive decline. By incorporating a diet rich in antioxidants, people can potentially lower their risk of cognitive impairment and support overall brain health. Oxidative stress is a process linked to neurodegenerative diseases like Alzheimer's.

Antioxidant-rich foods and beverages like green tea and moderate amounts of dark chocolate can further support brain health when consumed as part of a balanced diet. People can proactively support their cognitive health by including these foods and beverages in their daily meals. Colorful fruits and vegetables, such as blueberries, strawberries, and broccoli, are known for their high antioxidant content and not only offer protection against oxidative stress but also offer a variety of vitamins and minerals essential for brain function.

## THE VALUE AND SOURCES OF OMEGA-3 FATTY ACIDS

Omega-3 fatty acids are vital for brain health, especially when it comes to lowering inflammation and promoting cognitive function. These fats are mostly found in fatty fish, such as salmon, mackerel, and sardines, as well as in walnuts and flaxseeds. They are also important for preserving the structure and function of brain cells. Two types of omega-3 fatty acids, DHA and EPA, are especially beneficial because of their anti-inflammatory qualities and their role in neurotransmitter function, which has a positive impact on mood and cognition.

Omega-3 fatty acids can be added to the diet by eating fatty fish regularly—it can be baked, grilled, or added to salads and sandwiches. If you prefer plant-based sources, you can add ground flaxseeds to smoothies or oatmeal and have walnuts as a snack to get a rich source of alpha-linolenic acid (ALA), which is a precursor to

DHA and EPA. If your diet is deficient in omega-3s, you can take fish oil supplements, but make sure to speak with a physician for customized advice.

## VITAMIN AND MINERAL NEEDS FOR INDIVIDUALS WITH ALZHEIMER'S DISEASE

For Alzheimer's patients, meeting their vitamin and mineral needs is critical to maintaining overall health and cognitive function. Important nutrients include vitamin B12, which is found in animal products like meat, fish, and dairy, and vitamin D, which is obtained through sunshine exposure and fortified foods. Minerals like zinc and magnesium are found in foods like nuts, seeds, whole grains, and leafy green vegetables and play roles in neurotransmitter regulation.

A balanced diet that emphasizes a variety of nutrient-dense foods is the best way to guarantee that you are getting enough vitamins and minerals. You can also incorporate lean proteins, whole grains, and an abundance of fruits and vegetables into your meals to ensure that you are getting a wide range of essential nutrients. If you have any questions about how to customize your nutrient intake, speak with a registered dietitian or other healthcare provider. This is especially important if you have any dietary restrictions or difficulties with absorbing certain nutrients. Alzheimer's patients can improve their overall quality of life and cognitive health by emphasizing nutrient-rich foods and possibly taking supplements as directed by a doctor.

## THE IMPACT OF PROTEIN CONSUMPTION ON BRAIN ACTIVITY

Lean protein sources like chicken, fish, legumes, and tofu are excellent sources of protein and can help maintain cognitive abilities. Consumption of protein is important for brain function because it provides the building blocks for neurotransmitters, which help brain cells communicate with one another.

Amino acids, which make up proteins, are required for the synthesis of dopamine, serotonin, and other neurotransmitters that regulate mood, memory, and cognitive function.

To maximize the amount of protein that is consumed for brain function, try to incorporate foods high in protein into each meal and snack that you have throughout the day. You can also combine proteins with complex carbohydrates, like Greek yogurt with berries or hummus on whole-grain crackers, to support consistent energy levels and cognitive function. Processed meats and high-fat meats should be avoided as much as possible because they can cause inflammation and eventually impair brain health. Instead, people should prioritize lean, nutrient-dense sources of protein to support both brain health and general well-being.

## FIBER INCLUSION FOR IMPROVED DIGESTIVE HEALTH AND COGNITIVE ADVANTAGES

Fiber has two functions: it helps maintain healthy digestion and supports brain function. Soluble fiber, which is abundant in whole grains and vegetables, helps regulate blood sugar levels and supports healthy gut bacteria, which may influence brain health through the gut-brain axis. Insoluble fiber, on the other hand, is found in foods like apples, beans, and oats and supports regular bowel movements. Finally, it contributes to overall digestive health by reducing inflammation and promoting nutrient absorption.

Aim to consume a variety of fiber-rich foods throughout the day, including snacks like raw vegetables with hummus or whole fruit with nuts. Gradually increase fiber intake to avoid digestive discomfort, and drink plenty of water to support proper digestion and hydration. By maintaining a diet rich in both soluble and insoluble fiber, individuals can support digestive health and potentially enhance cognitive function over time. Whole, unprocessed foods such as fruits, vegetables, whole grains, and legumes are the best sources of fiber for the diet.

# CHAPTER FOUR

## STRATEGIES FOR MEAL PLANNING

### EASY WAYS TO PLAN MEALS FOR CAREGIVERS

Amid their demanding schedules, caregivers frequently struggle to provide nutritious meals that are also simple to prepare. This burden can be significantly reduced by making meal planning simpler. To start, make a weekly meal plan that consists of a variety of quick and easy recipes.

You may also want to batch-cook staples like grains, proteins, and vegetables so that you can mix and match them throughout the week. This method not only saves time but also guarantees that meals are balanced and nourishing.

Including the person with Alzheimer's disease as much as possible in meal preparation is another helpful tactic. This gives them a sense of independence and makes mealtime more interesting and pleasurable. You should also have a list of quick and easy recipes on hand, like one-pot meals or slow cooker dishes, which require little cleanup and can be customized to meet dietary needs.

Finally, to save time and minimize stress, take into consideration using meal delivery services or pre-made meal kits on occasion. These services offer balanced meals with little work on the part of caregivers, freeing them up to concentrate more on offering care and support. By using these helpful meal planning strategies, caregivers can make sure that they and their loved ones with Alzheimer's disease maintain a healthy and enjoyable eating routine.

**PREPARING EASY-TO-PREPARE, BALANCED MEALS**

Meal planning for people with Alzheimer's disease requires striking a balance between nutrition and ease of preparation. To start, include a range of vibrant fruits and vegetables in meals because they are high in vital vitamins and minerals. Choose lean proteins like chicken, fish, or beans because they are simple to cook and digest.

Whole grains like quinoa or brown rice offer fiber and long-lasting energy, which promotes general health.

Meal planning should focus on balancing carbohydrates, proteins, and healthy fats to support stable blood sugar levels and sustained energy throughout the day. Herbs and spices can be used to add flavor without using too much salt or sugar. Meals should be prepared in advance and kept in portioned containers to make serving quick and simple on busy days.

Furthermore, promote hydration by providing water throughout the day and including foods that are high in water content, such as soups, smoothies, or fruits. Caregivers can help their loved ones with Alzheimer's disease receive the essential nutrients they need while streamlining mealtime routines by concentrating on making balanced meals that are easy to prepare.

## CHANGING PORTION SIZES TO SUIT DIFFERENT APPETITES

Eating habits and preferences should be observed to determine appropriate portion sizes. Offer smaller, more frequent meals and snacks throughout the day to maintain energy levels and prevent overeating or undereating.

When caring for someone with Alzheimer's disease, it is imperative to adjust portion sizes according to individual appetites. Appetites can vary greatly depending on medication, activity levels, and overall health.

Offer nutrient-dense snacks like nuts, yogurt, or fresh fruit between meals to supplement nutritional intake without increasing overall portion sizes. Serve meals family-style, allowing people to serve themselves according to their appetite and preferences. Use smaller plates or bowls to visually cue appropriate portion sizes, making meals more manageable and less overwhelming.

Finally, work with medical professionals or dietitians to create customized nutrition plans that consider individual dietary requirements and preferences. Caregivers can support optimal nutrition and overall well-being for individuals with Alzheimer's disease by thoughtfully adjusting portion sizes and catering to individual appetites.

## SOME ADVICE FOR KEEPING MEAL SCHEDULES CONSISTENT

Establish regular meal times and adhere to them as much as possible to provide structure and predictability. Use visual cues, such as clocks or timers, to remind individuals of meal times and encourage them to participate in meal preparation or setting the table. Consistency in meal schedules is crucial in supporting individuals with Alzheimer's disease, as it helps regulate appetite, digestion, and overall well-being.

Keep a daily schedule that includes regular meal times, snacks, and hydration breaks to maintain energy levels and support overall health.

Reduce distractions like loud noises or crowded spaces to allow people to focus on eating and enjoying their food. Prepare meals in a calm and familiar environment to promote relaxation and reduce stress during meal times.

Caregivers can help individuals with Alzheimer's disease feel more stable and well-being by keeping a consistent meal schedule. They can also be more flexible and patient, understanding that meal schedules may need to be adjusted based on individual preferences or daily routines. Communicate with other caregivers or family members to ensure consistency in meal schedules, sharing responsibilities, and supporting each other in providing nutritious meals.

### INCLUDING VARIATION TO BOOST NUTRITIOUS CONSUMPTION

For people with Alzheimer's disease, adding diversity to meals is essential to improving nutritional intake and avoiding boredom. To start, rotate different protein sources, such as fish, poultry, eggs, or legumes, to offer a wide range of essential amino acids. Try different cooking techniques, such as grilling, baking, or steaming, to preserve flavors and nutrients.

Incorporate whole grains like oats, quinoa, or whole wheat pasta to add fiber and support digestive health. Offer dairy or dairy alternatives like yogurt or fortified plant-based milk to ensure adequate calcium intake for bone health. Incorporate a rainbow of colorful fruits and vegetables into meals to provide a wide range of vitamins, minerals, and antioxidants.

Encouraging people to try new foods or recipes can make mealtimes enjoyable and positive. Caregivers can ensure that their loved ones with Alzheimer's disease receive a well-rounded and nutritious diet by introducing new flavors and textures gradually, respecting individual preferences and dietary restrictions, and enhancing flavor with herbs, spices, or healthy sauces instead of relying too much on salt or sugar.

# SIMPLE AND FAST BREAKFAST RECIPES

## HEALTHY SMOOTHIE RECIPES TO GET YOU STARTED FAST

Smoothies can be made in a variety of ways to suit your taste and dietary requirements. For a nutritious smoothie, start with a base of leafy greens like spinach or kale for vitamins and minerals. Add fruits like berries, bananas, or mango for sweetness and extra vitamins.

Add ingredients like Greek yogurt, almond butter, or a plant-based protein powder to boost protein content. Finally, add a liquid like almond milk, coconut water, or regular water to create a creamy texture.

Blend a cup of frozen mango chunks, a ripe banana, a tablespoon of chia seeds, and a handful of spinach with coconut water to make a green smoothie. For a berry blast, combine mixed berries, a scoop of Greek yogurt, a handful of spinach, and a splash of almond milk; adjust sweetness with honey or dates if preferred. Pour into a glass and celebrate a revitalizing start to your day!

## EASY VARIATIONS FOR OATMEAL AND PORRIDGE

Breakfast staples like oatmeal and porridge are high in fiber and energy. Begin by cooking oats in water or milk until they reach your desired consistency. Use milk or almond milk for a creamy texture. Garnish your oatmeal with fresh fruit like banana slices or berries, nuts and seeds like almonds or chia seeds for crunch and healthy fats, and a drizzle of honey or maple syrup for sweetness. For a savory twist, top with avocado slices, poached egg, and cheese or herbs.

For a warm and cozy bowl of porridge, cook steel-cut oats with milk and water until thickened, and then stir in flavors like cinnamon and vanilla extract. Top with sliced apples and a sprinkle of cinnamon for a delicious start to your day!

To make overnight oats, combine rolled oats with milk, yogurt, and chia seeds in a jar or container. Let it sit in the fridge overnight, and in the morning, add toppings like nuts, seeds, and fruits!

## EGG-BASED RECIPES PACKED WITH VITAL NUTRIENTS

Eggs can be used for a variety of dishes and are a great source of protein, vitamins, and minerals. For a traditional breakfast, beat eggs with a little milk and cook in a nonstick pan until fluffy.

Top with cheese, chopped herbs, or diced vegetables for extra taste and nutrition. For a high-protein breakfast, beat eggs and add them to a heated pan with sautéed vegetables like spinach, bell peppers, and tomatoes.

Toast whole-grain bread, and top with avocado slices, cooked egg, and a dash of salt and pepper for a healthy breakfast sandwich. Whisk eggs with diced vegetables and pour into muffin tins; bake until set and enjoy these easy-to-transport breakfast bites all week long. Poached eggs can be served over whole-grain toast with sautéed greens for a filling and healthy way to start the day.

## BREAKFAST IDEAS THAT CAN BE APPLIED TO VARIOUS DIETS

Breakfast should be fun and can accommodate different diets. For vegetarians, try avocado toast with cherry tomatoes and feta cheese on top or a yogurt parfait with layers of Greek yogurt, granola, and fresh fruit. For vegans, try a smoothie bowl with blended fruits and nuts, seeds, and coconut flakes. For an even more satisfying breakfast, try overnight chia seed pudding with almond milk and berries on top.

For those on a low-carb diet, think about dishes like a spinach and feta omelet or Greek yogurt with nuts and seeds. Breakfast burritos made with scrambled eggs, black beans, and salsa wrapped in a lettuce leaf are another satisfying and low-carb option to fuel your morning. If you prefer a gluten-free breakfast, go for options like quinoa porridge cooked with almond milk and topped with sliced almonds and honey.

## SOME ADVICE FOR PROMOTING BREAKFAST CONSUMPTION

To sustain energy levels throughout the day, establish a morning routine. Begin by dedicating a specific time each morning to either prepare or grab a healthy breakfast. Make meal plans in advance by preparing ingredients or cooking larger batches of items, such as smoothie packs or overnight oats, which can be quickly assembled in the morning. Try a variety of flavors and textures to make breakfast engaging and pleasurable.

You can create a morning routine that supports health and vitality throughout the day by following these tips: Listen to your body's hunger cues and choose foods that satisfy your cravings while providing essential nutrients; Make breakfast a social occasion by sharing meals with family or friends whenever possible; Create a relaxing atmosphere by enjoying breakfast in a quiet space or outdoors to start your day on a positive note; and Stay hydrated by drinking water or herbal tea alongside your breakfast to support digestion and overall well-being.

# HEALTHY LUNCH AND DINNER SUGGESTIONS

## EASY-TO-DIGEST ONE-POT DINNERS

For people with Alzheimer's disease, making one-pot meals that are easy to digest is essential. These meals reduce preparation time and cleanup while making sure they are easy on the stomach. To begin, choose ingredients that are easily broken down, such as lean proteins like fish or chicken, and soft vegetables like carrots and zucchini. Whole grains, like brown rice or quinoa, are easier to break down than refined grains. To keep the dish flavorful and light, use low-sodium broth or water as a base.

To make these, just put all the ingredients into a big pot or slow cooker, cover, and simmer until everything is soft and cooked through. Season with herbs and spices instead of salt to add flavor without adding extra sodium. Stir occasionally to ensure that everything cooks evenly and to prevent sticking. Serve these warm to promote appetite and visual appeal.

These meals ensure that people with Alzheimer's disease receive a balanced, easily digestible meal that meets their nutritional needs, while also making cooking simpler.

## RICH IN NUTRIENT SOUPS AND STEWS

Lean proteins like beans, lentils, or diced chicken for added protein and texture. Nutrient-dense soups and stews are great options for Alzheimer's patients as they provide hydration, and essential nutrients, and are easy to consume. Start by choosing a variety of colorful vegetables like spinach, kale, tomatoes, and sweet potatoes, which are rich in vitamins, minerals, and antioxidants beneficial for brain health.

To make the soup or stew easier to swallow, chop the vegetables into bite-sized pieces to make them easier to chew and digest. Simmer the vegetables in a low-sodium broth with herbs and spices until they are tender. You can thin the soup or stew by adding extra broth or water as needed.

These high-nutrient soups and stews are great for supporting the dietary needs of Alzheimer's patients because they are comforting and warm, and they can be served with whole-grain bread or crackers on the side for extra crunch and fiber. Make sure the soup or stew is at a temperature that is safe to eat to avoid any discomfort.

**VEGETABLE-HEAVY SALADS WITH COMPONENTS THAT STRENGTHEN THE BRAIN**

For those suffering from Alzheimer's disease, colorful salads full of brain-boosting ingredients are a refreshing and nutritious option. Colorful veggies like broccoli, bell peppers, leafy greens, and cucumbers are high in vitamins and antioxidants that support brain function. You can also add healthy fats and crunch from walnuts, almonds, or seeds.

To make this dish easier to eat and digest, wash and cut the vegetables into bite-sized pieces. Then, combine them in a big bowl and dress them with simple vinaigrette that consists of olive oil, lemon juice, and herbs. If you want to make this dish a full meal, you can add lean proteins like tofu or grilled chicken.

These veggie-heavy salads are best served cold for maximum freshness and visual appeal. You may top them with a little cheese or fresh herbs if you'd like. These salads not only give Alzheimer's patients important nutrients, but they also help them stay hydrated and promote overall health.

**DINNERTIME MAIN DISHES PACKED WITH PROTEIN**

To guarantee that people with Alzheimer's disease get enough nutrition and keep their muscles strong, dinners must be high in protein. Lean protein sources, like baked or grilled fish, chicken, or tofu, are easy to chew and digest. Whole grains, like quinoa, brown rice, or whole wheat pasta, provide long-lasting energy and fiber.

To prepare, use herbs, spices, or marinade to add flavor without using a lot of salt; cook by grilling, baking, or sautéing in small amounts of oil to keep the food light and healthy; serve with roasted or steamed vegetables for extra vitamins and minerals.

Serve these protein-rich main dishes warm as part of a balanced dinner that meets the nutritional needs of Alzheimer's patients; make sure the servings are suitable, and chop the proteins into smaller pieces if needed to make chewing and swallowing easier.

## HOW TO ADJUST TEXTURES TO MAKE THEM EASIER TO SWALLOW AND CHEW

It is important to adjust textures to make eating and swallowing easier for people with Alzheimer's disease who may have trouble with these functions. To begin, choose foods that are easier to manage in the mouth, such as soft or finely chopped vegetables that are soft enough to mash with a fork, or lean meats that are soft enough to cut into smaller pieces.

For texture modification, puree foods like soups, stews, or cooked vegetables in a food processor or blender to create a smoother, easier-to-swallow consistency;

alternatively, mash foods like potatoes or avocados to a smooth texture or chop meats into bite-sized pieces.

Serve food at a moderate temperature to improve taste and comfort during meals. Make sure liquids are the right thickness to reduce choking hazards. Use thickening agents like cornstarch or commercial thickeners to change the consistency of soups, sauces, or beverages as needed.

Caregivers can support dietary needs and improve the dining experience for individuals living with Alzheimer's disease by appropriately modifying textures so that they can enjoy meals safely and comfortably that promote overall well-being and nutritional intake.

# SNACKS AND DRINKS TO REFUEL AND STAY HYDRATED

## OPTIONS FOR HEALTHFUL SNACKS TO KEEP YOUR ENERGY LEVELS UP

A healthy snack mix that combines complex carbs, protein, and healthy fats will sustain energy levels without spiking blood sugar. Some examples of such snacks are Greek yogurt with berries, whole-grain crackers with nut butter, or a small handful of nuts and seeds. These snacks offer a good balance of nutrients that support stable energy levels and help prevent fatigue.

Moreover, adding fruits and veggies to snacks can increase energy levels and supply vital vitamins and minerals. Some examples of such snacks are apple slices with cheese, carrot sticks with hummus, or a fruit smoothie with spinach. Snacking on these foods not only satisfies hunger but also supports a balanced diet, which is good for your overall health.

Nutritious snacks are especially important for people with Alzheimer's disease because they can be made ahead of time and kept in a convenient location, making it simple for them to access healthy options throughout the day. By emphasizing nutrient-dense ingredients and well-balanced combinations, both caregivers and individuals can support optimal energy levels and overall well-being.

**DRINKS THAT REHYDRATE AND PROMOTE COGNITIVE FUNCTION**

Hydrating beverages should not only quench thirst but also offer additional benefits for brain health. Herbal teas, which offer antioxidants and calming properties without caffeine, are a good option. Green tea, in particular, contains compounds that may support memory and brain function. Adequate hydration is crucial for cognitive function, especially for people with Alzheimer's disease.

Incorporating these beverages into daily routines can help individuals with Alzheimer's disease stay hydrated and support cognitive function. Another great option for hydration is coconut water, which replenishes electrolytes naturally and provides a mild sweetness without added sugars. It is low in calories and high in potassium, making it a refreshing option for maintaining hydration throughout the day.

Drinking hydrating beverages can help people with Alzheimer's disease stay hydrated and support cognitive function. These drinks can be consumed at any time of day and provide nutritional benefits in addition to hydration.

Caregivers can assist their loved ones in maintaining optimal hydration levels by selecting options that are low in sugar and caffeine-free.

## HOW TO MAKE HEALTHY SNACKS AT HOME

Caregivers can help individuals with Alzheimer's disease have access to healthy options throughout the day by making healthy snack preparations at home. To begin, choose recipes that are easy to make and use whole foods. Some ideas are energy balls made with oats, nut butter, and honey, or homemade trail mix with nuts and dried fruits.

Choose recipes that are easy to make in large quantities and store for later. Snacking is made easier when you portion it into individual servings, which not only saves time but also guarantees that you will always have snacks on hand when you're hungry. Caregivers can also maintain quality control over the ingredients they use by making their snacks, which can be customized to fit specific dietary requirements and dietary preferences.

By incorporating homemade snacks into a daily routine, caregivers can support overall well-being and provide individuals with Alzheimer's disease with nourishing options that promote health and enjoyment. Homemade snacks can be customized to include ingredients that support brain health, such as nuts, seeds, and antioxidant-rich fruits. These snacks provide essential nutrients while minimizing processed sugars and unhealthy fats.

## SNACK IDEAS TO CONTROL YOUR APPETITE IN BETWEEN MEALS

For people with Alzheimer's disease, controlling hunger in between meals is critical to maintaining stable energy levels and preventing overindulgence. Nutrient-dense, satisfying snacks to eat in between meals include whole fruits (apples, bananas, etc.) with nut butter or yogurt with granola and berries; these combinations provide a good balance of carbohydrates, protein, and healthy fats.

Caregivers can guarantee that individuals with Alzheimer's disease have wholesome snacks available throughout the day by planning and making simple snacks that require little preparation, like pre-cut vegetables with hummus or cheese slices with whole-grain crackers. These snacks can be portioned in advance and kept in handy containers for easy access.

Caregivers can support the overall health and well-being of individuals with Alzheimer's disease by providing balanced snack options.

Sugary snacks and processed foods can cause fluctuations in blood sugar levels and contribute to overeating. Instead, choose snacks that promote satiety and provide essential nutrients.

**REASONS WHY MINDFUL EATING IS IMPORTANT FOR ALZHEIMER'S PATIENTS**

For people with Alzheimer's disease, mindful eating can improve the enjoyment of meals and snacks while promoting awareness of hunger and fullness cues. It involves encouraging people to eat slowly, savoring each bite, and focusing on the flavors and textures of food.

Mindful eating is about paying attention to the sensory experience of food, including taste, texture, and aroma.

Additionally, caregivers can support nutritional intake and general well-being by being present during meals and snacks; they can also help individuals with Alzheimer's disease maintain healthy eating habits and avoid overeating; and they can promote mindfulness and enjoyment of food by providing a peaceful, welcoming, distraction-free environment for meals.

Caregivers can support nutritional intake and overall health by emphasizing mindful eating practices. Include comfort foods and favorite foods in meals and snacks to increase comfort and satisfaction. Respect dietary preferences and accommodate individual tastes to create a positive eating experience.

# CHAPTER FIVE

## RECIPES FOR SPECIAL OCCASIONS AND HOLIDAYS

### FESTIVE RECIPES

Nutritious and enjoyable recipes can be made by concentrating on whole, fresh ingredients that are high in nutrients. For instance, you can use seasonal fruits and vegetables in dishes like roasted butternut squash with herbs or a vibrant salad with berries and nuts. These dishes will not only bring color and vital nutrients to your holiday table, but they will also provide you with plenty of vitamins and minerals.

An alternative strategy is to look into lean protein options, which are lighter than traditional holiday meats. Examples of these include baked fish with a citrus glaze or grilled turkey breast.

These proteins can be paired with whole grains, like quinoa pilaf or wild rice stuffing, to create a well-rounded meal that promotes overall and brain health.

And last, remember to incorporate heart-healthy fats from foods like nuts, avocados, and olive oil into your recipes. These fats can support cognitive function and give food a satisfying texture. By emphasizing nutrient-dense ingredients and flavorful combinations, you can make delicious, scrumptious, and Alzheimer's disease-friendly holiday meals.

## HOW TO MODIFY TRADITIONAL DISHES FOR DIETARY NEEDS

Changing traditional dishes to suit dietary requirements requires careful substitution and adjustment of ingredients without compromising flavor or texture. For example, you can reduce the saturated fat content of mashed potatoes by using Greek yogurt or low-fat milk in place of heavy cream, while maintaining the creamy texture. Similarly, you can increase the fiber and nutrient content of baking recipes by using almond flour or whole wheat flour in place of refined white flour.

To increase flavor without adding extra sodium, try cutting back on salt by using herbs and spices like thyme, rosemary, and garlic powder. You may also try minimizing the amount of added sugar in sweets by using natural sweeteners like honey or maple syrup, which will still satisfy your sweet craving.

As part of an Alzheimer's disease diet, it's critical to emphasize foods high in nutrients that promote brain health. Adding vibrant veggies, lean proteins, and healthy fats to modified dishes can enhance overall health while respecting traditional flavors and cooking methods.

## DESSERTS WITH BRAIN-BOOSTING INGREDIENTS

Using ingredients like dark chocolate, which is high in antioxidants and may improve blood flow to the brain, can be a delicious way to support cognitive function during special occasions. Try making a dark chocolate mousse with avocado for extra creaminess and heart-healthy fats.

Berries: Packed with vitamins and antioxidants that support brain function, berries like blueberries, strawberries, or raspberries can also be a great addition to your dessert table. Try serving them as a topping for yogurt parfaits or as a refreshing fruit salad to bring some natural sweetness and eye-catching colors.

Nuts like walnuts and almonds are also great sources of vitamin E and omega-3 fatty acids, which are thought to support cognitive function. You can incorporate nuts into dessert recipes like almond flour cookies or nutty granola bars for a tasty and nutritious treat.

Desserts with components that support brain function can be made to provide sweet ends to meals that support overall satisfaction and well-being for people on an Alzheimer's disease diet.

## CREATING A COMFORTING MEAL ENVIRONMENT FOR HOLIDAYS

Creating a comfortable meal environment for holidays can improve the dining experience for people with Alzheimer's disease. To begin, create a calm and stress-relieving atmosphere with soft lighting and relaxing music. During meals, use utensils and familiar tableware that are easy for people with cognitive impairments to grasp and use.

To promote social connection and avoid overpowering sensory experiences, think about serving meals family-style or in smaller amounts. Set up seats to encourage conversation and reduce distractions, including crowded areas or loud noises, which can ruin the fun of mealtimes.

Bring cozy scents into the kitchen by using herbs like cinnamon or rosemary, which can arouse fond memories and increase appetite. Provide options when it is feasible to meet dietary restrictions and individual tastes so that everyone feels welcomed and appreciated over the holidays.

You may encourage a feeling of comfort and satisfaction for people with Alzheimer's disease by making your dining area cozy and welcoming. This will improve their overall quality of life and dining experience.

## TIPS FOR INCLUDING ALZHEIMER'S PATIENTS IN MEAL PREPARATION

Assigning basic tasks like washing vegetables or stirring ingredients can help individuals feel included and contribute to the meal preparation process. Including Alzheimer's patients in meal preparation can be a meaningful and engaging activity that encourages independence and social interaction.

Focus on safe and manageable activities, modifying tasks based on individual skills and preferences to provide a good experience. Provide clear and concise directions, demonstrating each step as needed to assist understanding and participation.

Cooking together can increase cognitive function and develop a sense of connection with loved ones during dinner preparation. To that end, encourage conversation and nostalgia by talking about favorite recipes, culinary memories, and family customs.

Last but not least, be kind and understanding during the process, providing help when needed but letting people keep their sense of pride and accomplishment in making holiday meals. By getting Alzheimer's patients involved in meal preparation, you can create experiences that are meaningful and improve their quality of life in general.

Simplifying the process of cooking holiday meals, adjusting classic recipes, developing brain-boosting desserts, creating cozy dining spaces, and including Alzheimer's patients in meal preparation are all possible with these strategies. All of them center around doable actions that guarantee satisfying eating experiences that promote both physical and mental well-being.

# CHAPTER SIX

## COOKING TRICKS AND STRATEGIES FOR SENIORS

## SETTING UP THE KITCHEN TO MAKE MEAL PREPARATION EASIER

The kitchen is a vital space for caregivers of Alzheimer's patients to prepare meals efficiently. Begin by clearing out countertops and cabinets to make room for a clear workspace. Keep frequently used items close at hand to reduce the need for extensive searching. Combine similar items, like cookware and utensils, to expedite the cooking process. Label shelves and containers clearly to help identify tools and ingredients quickly.

A color-coded system for labeling foods based on their expiration dates can be implemented to prevent spoilage and ensure safety. Regularly review and update the organization system to accommodate changing needs and preferences. Consider setting up dedicated stations for different meal preparation stages, such as a chopping area with accessible knives and cutting boards.

## FLEXIBLE KITCHEN UTENSILS AND APPLIANCES

Caretakers of people with Alzheimer's disease can greatly simplify meal preparation by selecting ergonomic, lightweight utensils with non-slip grips to improve control and lessen strain on hands and wrists; choose knives with safety features like easy-grip handles and blade guards to reduce the chance of cuts; and use automatic appliances like food processors and electric can openers to simplify tasks requiring strength or precision.

Install grab bars near sinks and cooking areas to offer extra stability and support. Consider using utensils and gadgets made specifically for Alzheimer's patients, like easy-grip cups and adaptive eating utensils. Make sure all equipment is accessible and well-maintained to encourage independence and confidence during meal preparation. Adjust countertops and tables to accommodate wheelchair users or people with mobility challenges.

## HOW TO BE PATIENT WHEN FACING COOKING DIFFICULTIES

Caregivers of individuals with Alzheimer's disease must be patient when addressing cooking challenges. Start by creating a peaceful and comforting environment, reducing noise and disruptions.

Divide complicated recipes into smaller, more manageable steps, giving clear directions and examples as needed. Encourage the person to help prepare meals at their own pace, offering support and encouragement along the way.

Be flexible and adaptable in your approach, modifying recipes and techniques based on the patient's capabilities and comfort level. Allow extra time for meal preparation to accommodate delays or interruptions, maintaining a relaxed and stress-free atmosphere. Celebrate small successes and milestones to boost morale and foster a positive cooking experience for both caregiver and patient.

Engage in active listening and watch out for non-verbal cues to understand the individual's preferences and limitations.

## ADVICE FOR PROMOTING SELF-SUFFICIENCY IN MEAL PREPARATION

Encouraging independence in meal tasks for Alzheimer's patients improves their quality of life and their sense of self. Start by letting them plan and shop for their meals, letting them select their favorite foods and ingredients.

Make recipes simpler and use pictures and step-by-step instructions to make it easier for them to understand and participate. Give them small tasks to do, like stirring ingredients or setting the table, so they feel like they've accomplished something.

Adaptive strategies, like pre-measured ingredients and portioned serving utensils, can promote independence while ensuring safety and consistency. Establish a supportive environment that encourages experimentation and creativity in meal preparation. Offer choices whenever possible, respecting individual preferences and dietary restrictions. Provide positive reinforcement and praise for efforts, regardless of the outcome, to build confidence and motivation.

## SAFETY STEPS TO AVOID MISHAPS IN THE KITCHEN

When caring for patients with Alzheimer's disease, it is imperative to put safety precautions in place to prevent accidents in the kitchen. To start, store potentially dangerous items, like sharp knives and cleaning supplies, in locked cabinets or drawers. Use childproof locks on oven and stove controls to prevent accidental use. Keep workspaces clear of clutter and clear of paths to minimize the risk of trips and falls.

To improve visibility and stability when preparing meals, install non-slip flooring and bright lighting. Keep an eye out for signs of confusion or distraction when supervising cooking activities. Discuss safety procedures with family members and caregivers and keep emergency contact information close at hand.

Promote the use of oven mitts and pot holders to prevent burns and scalds.

Caregivers can efficiently manage meal preparation while enabling adults with Alzheimer's disease to preserve a sense of autonomy and dignity. Some strategies to consider include emphasizing organization, implementing adapted tools, encouraging patience, promoting independence, and assuring safety.

# CHAPTER SEVEN

## TAKING CARE OF EATING CHALLENGES AND DIETARY ADJUSTMENTS

### RECOGNIZING TYPICAL EATING CHALLENGES IN ALZHEIMER'S PATIENTS

Alzheimer's disease can cause a variety of eating difficulties that caregivers and family members must recognize and effectively manage. For example, people with the disease may have trouble identifying food or utensils, which can cause confusion and frustration when it comes to mealtimes. They may also experience changes in appetite, such as decreased hunger or increased cravings for particular foods, which can make meal planning and nutrition management more difficult.

In addition, individuals with Alzheimer's disease may experience difficulties with motor skills, which can make it difficult for them to chew food or use utensils correctly.

This can lead to longer meal times or an inability to finish meals, which can affect overall nutrition intake. As the disease advances, people may also lose the ability to communicate their food preferences or recognize hunger cues, which calls for a more intuitive method of meal planning and serving.

To maintain nutritional health and improve the quality of life for Alzheimer's patients, caregivers should be aware of these challenges and modify mealtime strategies accordingly. This may entail simplifying the dining environment, using adaptive utensils if necessary, and showing patience and support during mealtimes.

## HOW TO HANDLE TASTE AND APPETITE SHIFTS

Alzheimer's disease patients frequently experience changes in taste and appetite, which can have a substantial impact on eating habits. Patients may become more interested in sweeter foods or lose interest in meals they used to enjoy because of altered taste perceptions.

Caregivers can help patients with these changes by introducing new flavors and textures that they find appealing.

Small, frequent meals throughout the day can help maintain adequate nutrition intake, even if appetite fluctuates. Mealtime enjoyment can also be increased by offering familiar foods and avoiding overwhelming flavors or complicated dishes. It's important to provide a variety of nutritious options while respecting personal choices.

Caregivers should also keep an eye on food intake and modify meal plans in response to feedback and observations. Speaking with a medical expert or dietitian who specializes in Alzheimer's care can offer insightful advice and individualized dietary recommendations. Caregivers can help Alzheimer's patients maintain better nutritional health by sensitively and creatively adjusting to changes in appetite and taste.

## ADVICE FOR ENCOURAGING SATISFYING MEAL EXPERIENCES

Encouraging mealtimes for Alzheimer's patients is critical to their overall health and dietary intake. To begin, create a peaceful, comfortable dining space free of noise and distractions. Use dishes and cutlery that the patient is familiar with to ease confusion and improve comfort.

Bring people together for meals as a family or with friends to foster social interaction and stimulate appetite and a positive mealtime atmosphere. Adding favorite foods and visually appealing, colorful dishes can also pique people's interest and stimulate appetite.

Additionally, think about scheduling meals to align with the person's preferred times of day and refrain from rushing through meal preparation and serving. Flexibility and patience are essential in fostering positive meal experiences, enabling Alzheimer's patients to eat in a relaxed environment and at their own pace.

## MODIFYING RECIPES TO ADDRESS CHEWING AND SWALLOWING CHALLENGES

Alzheimer's patients may find it difficult to chew and swallow food, which can make it dangerous for them to eat solid food. To help patients with these challenges, caregivers can adjust recipes to make food easier to chew and swallow. This can involve cooking vegetables until they are soft or pureeing meals to a smoother consistency.

Reduce the risk of choking or discomfort during meals by avoiding tough or hard-to-chew foods like raw vegetables or tough chunks of meat. Using ground meats or adding yogurt and sauces can also help moisten dishes, making them easier to swallow.

Caregivers can make sure that meals are safe and enjoyable for Alzheimer's patients by modifying recipes thoughtfully and proactively. Serving smaller portions and encouraging slower eating can also help manage chewing and swallowing difficulties. It's important to consult with a healthcare professional or speech therapist for specific dietary recommendations and techniques tailored to the individual's needs.

## COLLABORATING WITH MEDICAL EXPERTS TO PROVIDE NUTRITIONAL ADVICE

Working with healthcare professionals who specialize in geriatric care and nutrition can help you navigate the challenges and changes in diet that come with Alzheimer's disease. They can offer important advice on meal planning strategies, adaptive eating techniques, and nutritional requirements.

In addition to providing insights into managing medication interactions that may affect appetite or taste perceptions, speaking with a dietitian can help caregivers create customized meal plans that meet individual dietary needs and preferences while guaranteeing adequate nutrition intake.

Regular consultations with healthcare professionals enable caregivers to stay informed about the latest research and best practices in Alzheimer's nutrition, empowering them to make informed decisions for optimal dietary management. Additionally, speech therapists can offer techniques to improve chewing and swallowing abilities, ensuring that meals are safe and comfortable for patients with Alzheimer's disease.

Caregivers can improve the nutritional health and quality of diet for Alzheimer's patients by collaborating with medical specialists. This will improve the patient's general health and quality of life.

# CHAPTER EIGHT

## COMMON QUESTIONS AND EXTENSIVE ANSWERS

### TAKING CARE OF NUTRITIONAL ISSUES PARTICULAR TO ALZHEIMER'S PATIENTS

A balanced diet rich in nutrients can help manage symptoms and slow the progression of the disease. When it comes to Alzheimer's patients, nutrition is critical to maintaining overall health and cognitive function.

You should emphasize including foods that are good for the brain, such as leafy greens, berries, fatty fish rich in omega-3 fatty acids, and nuts. These foods provide vital vitamins, antioxidants, and healthy fats that support brain health and reduce inflammation.

Caregivers need to emphasize hydration because individuals with Alzheimer's disease may forget to drink water, which increases the risk of dehydration. Offer water, herbal teas, and foods that are high in water content, such as fruits and soups, to help stabilize blood sugar levels and sustain energy levels throughout the day.

To ensure that nutritional needs are met while accommodating chewing and swallowing difficulties, meal plans should be customized based on the individual's preferences, dietary restrictions, and stage of Alzheimer's disease; regular mealtimes in a familiar and calm setting can also help with digestion. Speak with a registered dietitian for more information.

## HOW TO MANAGE NUTRITIONAL ADJUSTMENTS AS ALZHEIMER'S ADVANCES

As Alzheimer's disease advances, dietary requirements, and eating habits may also change, necessitating modifications to guarantee appropriate nutrition and comfort. Keep an eye on eating habits and preferences, modifying meals to accommodate changing tastes and capacities. If chewing becomes difficult, consider soft or pureed foods; additionally, provide small, frequent meals or snacks to sustain energy levels all day.

As much as possible, involve the person in meal preparation to foster independence and enjoyment in food-related activities. Make choices simpler to avoid confusion and overwhelm by providing recognizable foods that are simple to recognize and eat. Use verbal cues and visual cues to assist with eating, making sure meals smell good and look good.

Encourage regular physical activity as part of a healthy routine, as this can stimulate appetite and improve overall well-being. Seek support from healthcare professionals or nutrition experts for guidance on adapting diets as Alzheimer's symptoms change. Maintain a calm dining environment free from distractions, loud noises, or crowded spaces to promote relaxation and focus during meals.

### STRATEGIES FOR HANDLING WEIGHT GAIN OR LOSS

Changes in appetite, metabolism, and physical activity levels can all contribute to weight changes in people with Alzheimer's disease. It is important to keep a regular eye on weight and speak with healthcare professionals as soon as concerns arise. A healthy weight maintenance strategy is to emphasize nutrient-dense foods that supply vital vitamins and minerals without adding unnecessary calories.

Offer snacks or small meals throughout the day to boost calorie intake if weight loss is a concern; if weight gain becomes an issue, prioritize portion control and mindful eating practices, emphasizing balanced meals and healthy snacks. Regular physical activity, appropriate to the individual's abilities and preferences, can help regulate appetite, improve muscle tone, and support overall health.

Establish a welcoming dining space that promotes stress reduction and decreases eating behaviors related to stress. Work with healthcare professionals to address underlying factors that contribute to weight fluctuations, such as medication side effects or underlying medical conditions. Modify meal plans to accommodate evolving dietary requirements and support healthy weight management as the disease progresses.

## RECOGNIZING SUPPLEMENTS' SIGNIFICANCE IN ALZHEIMER'S DIET

When it comes to Alzheimer's nutrition, supplements can help by providing extra nutrients that may be lost through reduced appetite or difficulty eating. Before beginning any new supplement regimen, speak with a healthcare provider to make sure it's safe and suitable for the patient's condition and current medications. Supplements that support brain health, like omega-3 fatty acids, vitamin E, and B vitamins, have been shown to have potential benefits for cognitive function.

When selecting supplements, take into account the person's dietary intake, trying to supplement rather than replace whole foods; seek out high-quality supplements from reliable manufacturers to ensure purity and effectiveness; keep an eye out for any negative effects or interactions with medications; and adjust dosages as advised by healthcare professionals.

To support overall health and well-being, incorporate supplements into a comprehensive nutrition plan that includes a variety of nutrient-rich foods. Inform family members and caregivers about the significance of supplement routine adherence and consistency to promote long-term benefits for cognitive function and quality of life in Alzheimer's disease patients.

## RESPONSES TO COMMON QUESTIONS CONCERNING THE ALZHEIMER'S DIET

Concerns about Alzheimer's diet, including managing eating disorders, providing appropriate hydration, and supporting brain health through diet are common among families and caregivers. It is important to provide fluids throughout the day, such as water and hydrating foods like fruits and soups, to prevent dehydration risks common in Alzheimer's patients who may forget to drink.

To address eating challenges, meal textures and sizes should be adjusted as necessary, with an emphasis on familiar foods that are simple to identify and eat. People should be involved in meal preparation and dining experiences to increase enjoyment and independence, as well as to create a distraction-free, relaxed environment. Registered dietitians or healthcare professionals can provide individualized nutrition plans that take into account dietary preferences and Alzheimer's stage of progression.

To promote overall health and quality of life through mindful nutrition and supportive caregiving practices, it is important to educate caregivers about the importance of balanced nutrition, which includes brain-healthy foods like berries, leafy greens, and fatty fish rich in omega-3s. These foods provide essential nutrients that support cognitive function and overall well-being. Regular physical activity and social engagement should also be encouraged.

www.ingramcontent.com/pod-product-compliance
Lightning Source LLC
Chambersburg PA
CBHW071839210526
45479CB00001B/206